What Is Sex

A Comprehensive Guide to Sex Education, Exploring Pleasure and Self-Discovery, Navigating Sexual Wellness and Relationships and Creating Safe and Empowering Spaces for Sexual Learning

Cheryl Bach

What Is Sex

Cheryl Bach

Table of Contents

Chapter 1

Introduction to Sex Education and the Importance of Comprehensive, Inclusive Education

A. Explanation of Key Terms and Concepts

Sex education is defined as the process of acquiring information and forming attitudes and beliefs related to sex, sexuality, relationships, and sexual health. It is important to note that sex education does not solely focus on sexual activity but also includes many aspects related to body and mental development.

Some key terms covered in this chapter include:

What Is Sex

Consent: permission given for something to happen, in particular sexual activity.

Contraception: methods used to prevent unwanted pregnancy and the spread of sexually transmitted infections.

Sexual Orientation/Identity: for whom individuals feel attraction towards - heterosexual, homosexual, bisexual etc., and how one identifies oneself as in relation to these attractions.

Gender Identity: the internal sense of being male, female/non-binary, or other gender categories different from the one assigned at birth.

B. Brief History of Sex Education in the U.S.

Sex education in the United States has a long and complex history. In the early 1900s, sex education focused primarily on the prevention of sexually transmitted infections (STIs). This approach was limited, however, and often relied on shaming and scare tactics to discourage sexual activity.

It wasn't until the 1960s and 1970s that sex education began to focus more on comprehensive education that included topics such as contraception, communication skills, and relationship dynamics. However, this was met with backlash and controversy, with some communities expressing that this kind of education was inappropriate for young people.

Despite increased efforts to provide comprehensive sex education in schools, there remains inconsistency in what is being taught across the country. Many states still prioritize abstinence-only education over comprehensive education, which can leave young people vulnerable to unintended pregnancies, STIs, and unhealthy relationships.

What Is Sex

C. Overview of What Will Be Covered in the Book

This book aims to provide a comprehensive guide to sex education, exploring pleasure and self-discovery, navigating sexual wellness and relationships, and creating safe and empowering spaces for sexual learning.

The topics covered in this book will include:

Sexual Anatomy and Physiology: A detailed overview of the male and female reproductive systems, what they do, and how they function.

Sexual Health and Wellness: Discussions on sexual challenges such as sexual dysfunction, STIs/STDs, sexual self-care, emotional and psychological well-being.

Sexual Relationships and Communication: Guidance on navigating different types of relationships, the importance of consent and communication, and strategies for fostering healthy sexual relationships.

Empowerment and Advocating for Inclusive Spaces: Exploration of the power dynamics involved in sexual relationships, how to identify and address issues of sexual harassment and violence, and how to advocate for creating safe spaces for all around sexual education.

Understanding Sexual Diversity: Discussions on different sexual orientations, gender identities, and the importance of accepting and respecting diverse experiences.

Navigating Sexual Intimacy and Pleasure: Discussions on sexual pleasure, masturbation, and how to navigate self-exploration with confidence and safety.

Digital sex and Education: A detailed exploration of digital technologies that have shaped contemporary sexuality like sexting, pornography, social media, and other digital mediums on individuals and society as a whole.

Spiritual and ritual perspectives on sexuality: Examination of cultural and spiritual perspectives on sexuality, how spirituality can influence one's approach to sexuality and ways to incorporate sexuality into spiritual practices.

Conclusion and Reflections: Final reflections on what has been covered throughout the book, a summary of key takeaways, and suggestions for further learning and exploration.

Overall, this book seeks to provide a comprehensive and inclusive guide to sex education that empowers readers to explore their sexuality safely and confidently. By providing accurate information, promoting self-reflection, and fostering empathy, this book aims to create spaces where readers feel safe and free to explore and express their sexual selves.

What Is Sex

Chapter II

Navigating Personal and Cultural Discoveries around Sexuality

A. Understanding Individual Sexual Preferences and Desires

When it comes to sexuality, there is no normal or one-size-fits-all approach. Every individual has unique desires and preferences that can change over time. It is important to understand and respect our own sexual preferences and desires without judgment or shame.

Exploring sexuality can be a process of self-discovery that includes experimenting with different sexual experiences, learning from mistakes, and embracing what feels authentic.

What Is Sex

Acknowledging our own unique sexual preferences can help us cultivate healthy sexual relationships with partners who share similar desires and enable communication to express what we want from those partnerships.

B. Challenging Cultural and Societal Attitudes towards Sexuality

Cultural and societal attitudes towards sexuality shape our perspectives and attitudes towards what is positive and acceptable. Unfortunately, many of these attitudes can be harmful, perpetuating shame, judgment, and stigma around sexuality and sexual expression. It is important for individuals to challenge these societal attitudes and embrace a positive attitude towards sexuality.

For example, there may be societal pressures to conform to traditional gender roles or expectations of what is considered "normal" when it comes to sexual desires and preferences. These attitudes can limit an individual's exploration of their own sexuality and make them feel isolated and alienated from others who express preferences outside the norms. Challenging these ideas empowers individuals to be open and honest about their sexuality and helps combat existing stigmas.

C. Addressing Common Myths and Misconceptions

There are many myths and misconceptions about sexuality that still exist today. These commonly perpetuated beliefs can have a harmful impact on how individuals perceive and approach their own sexualities.

Some common myths around sexuality include the belief that men have a higher sexual drive or desire, that sex should always lead to orgasm, and that individuals with certain gender identities or sexual orientations are abnormal or deviant. It is important to address and debunk these myths to create a more accurate and understanding view of sexuality.

What Is Sex

For instance, everyone has different sexual desires, regardless of gender, and there is no right or wrong way to approach sex. Orgasm is not the ultimate goal of sexual experience, and it's important to prioritize feelings of intimacy and pleasure over achieving that goal. Furthermore, individuals who identify with certain gender identities or sexual orientations are just as valid as anyone else, and their experiences should not be stigmatized or invalidated by societal norms.

By addressing common myths and misconceptions around sexuality, individuals can combat harmful attitudes and better understand and embrace their own unique sexual desires and preferences. This can lead to a more positive and empowering approach to sexuality that prioritizes healthy communication and respect between partners.

Cheryl Bach

In conclusion, navigating personal and cultural discoveries around sexuality is an essential aspect of developing a healthy and positive approach to sex education. By understanding and respecting our own unique sexual desires and challenging harmful societal attitudes and beliefs, we can create safe and empowering spaces for learning and exploration.

Addressing common myths and misconceptions around sexuality enables individuals to better understand and embrace their own sexualities and cultivate healthy relationships with partners who share similar desires. Ultimately, by fostering a more accurate and accepting cultural understanding of sexuality, we can promote positive attitudes towards sexual wellness and self-discovery.

What Is Sex

Chapter III

Exploration of Different Sexual Interest and Desires

A. Explanation of a Wide Range of Sexual Experiences

Sexuality is diverse and multifaceted, with a wide range of sexual experiences and desires. Understanding different sexual preferences is essential in creating safe and inclusive spaces for individuals to explore and express their sexuality.

Some examples of sexual experiences include heterosexual, homosexual, bisexual, demisexual, asexual, pansexual, and queer. Each of these identities represents a unique approach to sexual attraction and desire. Understanding and respecting these different experiences is important for creating an inclusive and accepting community that celebrates diversity.

B. Explanation of Diverse Sexual Identities

Sexual identity encompasses many aspects of life, including race, gender identity, and socio-economic status. Intersectionality is a concept that recognizes that individuals have multiple identities that intersect and influence each other, leading to unique and complex experiences.

For example, people of color and those who identify as LGBTQIA+ may face additional barriers and stigma when exploring and expressing their sexuality. Transgender individuals may also face discrimination and marginalization when it comes to sexual expression.

Cheryl Bach

It is essential to understand and respect the diverse identities that influence sexual experiences and work towards creating supportive and inclusive environments for all individuals to explore and express their sexuality without fear or judgment.

C. Discussion of Sexual Attraction and Common Stereotypes and Stigmas

Sexual attraction is a complex and individual experience that can be influenced by a range of factors, including personality, physical appearance, and emotional connection. However, many common stereotypes and stigmas continue to persist around attraction, including beliefs that certain sexual orientations are abnormal or that individuals have control over their attractions.

It is important to challenge these stereotypes and stigmas and instead recognize that sexual attraction is a personal and uncontrollable experience that should be respected and celebrated, regardless of orientation. Additionally, attraction should not be conflated with harmful behaviors such as harassment or sexual assault, and it is important to address and prevent these behaviors in all communities.

By creating a more accepting and inclusive environment that values individual experiences and perspectives, we can foster a culture that promotes healthy and respectful sexual expression. This involves challenging outdated stereotypes and stigmas and embracing a diversity of sexual identities and experiences.

Chapter IV

Comprehensive Overview of Sexual Health and Wellness

A. Comprehensive Overview of Sexual Anatomy, Physiology, and Health

Sexual anatomy includes the physical structures and organs that are involved in sexual experience, such as the genitals and reproductive system. Understanding the physiology of these structures is essential for maintaining sexual health and well-being.

For instance, the female reproductive system includes the ovaries, uterus, and vagina, while the male reproductive system includes the testes, prostate, and penis. Additionally, the neural pathways and chemical processes that influence sexual desire and arousal are complex and still not fully understood by science. By developing a comprehensive understanding of sexual anatomy and physiology, individuals can make informed decisions about their sexual well-being.

B. Exploring Challenges with Sexual Health

Unfortunately, sexual dysfunctions, sexually transmitted diseases, and illnesses are common challenges that individuals may face when it comes to maintaining sexual health. Sexual dysfunctions can include problems with arousal, orgasm, or desire, and can impact individuals of all genders and sexual orientations. Additionally, sexually transmitted infections (STIs) and diseases (STDs) are a major concern due to their prevalence and potential long-term health consequences.

Cheryl Bach

It is important to practice safe sex and undergo regular STI testing to prevent the spread of infections and ensure optimal health outcomes. There are also several treatment options available for individuals who may be experiencing sexual dysfunctions, including therapy, medication, and lifestyle changes.

C. Discussion of Sexual Self-Care

Sexual self-care is an essential element of overall sexual wellness and involves taking care of one's emotional, psychological, and physical well-being. This can include practicing self-compassion and self-love, engaging in stress-reducing activities, and developing a healthy relationship with sexuality.

In addition to these practices, it is important to prioritize emotional and psychological well-being, such as identifying and addressing negative thought patterns or beliefs around sexuality. This can also involve processing past traumas or experiences related to sexuality and developing strategies to cope with anxiety or depression.

Engaging in healthy sexual relationships is also a crucial aspect of sexual self-care. This involves having open and honest communication with partners, respecting boundaries, and prioritizing consent and safety.

By promoting comprehensive education about sexual health and wellness, we can create safe and empowering spaces for individuals to explore their sexuality. This includes destigmatizing sexual challenges and dysfunctions and providing resources for individuals to access support and care. Ultimately, prioritizing sexual education and wellness can lead to greater sexual satisfaction, healthier relationships, and overall well-being.

Chapter V

Sexual Relationships and Communication

A. A Comprehensive Guide on Navigating Different Relationships

Navigating different types of sexual relationships, such as monogamy, polyamory, and open relationships, can be complex and nuanced. Each relationship type has its unique challenges and benefits and requires informed consent and communication from all parties involved.

When it comes to monogamous relationships, it is crucial to establish clear boundaries and expectations around sexual exclusivity. Polyamory and open relationships require even more open and honest communication to ensure that all parties involved are on the same page. This includes setting boundaries around physical and emotional intimacy, practicing safe sex, and ongoing communication about each individual's needs and desires.

B. Importance of Consent and Communication in a Healthy Sexual Relationship

Consent and communication are two fundamental aspects of building healthy sexual relationships. Consent involves giving explicit permission for any sexual activity, and requires individuals to be fully informed and engaged in the decision-making process. Communication involves open and honest dialogue about boundaries, expectations, desires, and concerns.

When it comes to consent, it is essential to respect and value the opinions and comfort of all parties involved. An enthusiastic 'yes' is the only acceptable response for sexual activity; otherwise, it's considered a 'no'. Consent can and should be revoked at any time during sexual activity.

Communication is also paramount - healthy sexual relationships require individuals to openly communicate their wants and needs, as well as any concerns or reservations. This can involve sharing fantasies or desires, expressing boundaries or limitations, asking for feedback, and checking in with partners.

C. Strategies for Fostering Healthy Sexual Relationships

Developing healthy sexual relationships can take time and effort, but there are several strategies that can promote supportive and empowering sexual experiences. Firstly, establishing clear boundaries and expectations is essential for feeling secure and respected in a sexual relationship. This includes discussing preferred forms of sexual activity, preferred levels of intimacy, and any potential limitations or restrictions.

Secondly, ongoing communication is vital for maintaining a healthy sexual relationship. This involves checking in with partners regularly about their wants, needs, and any changes in boundaries or expectations. Being willing to listen without judgment or defensiveness can help ensure that all parties feel heard and valued.

Thirdly, promoting safe sex practices is important for creating a supportive and empowering sexual environment. This can involve discussing STI testing and prevention methods, including using condoms or other forms of protection, and regular testing.

Finally, it is essential to prioritize mutual respect and empathy in a sexual relationship. This includes respecting and valuing partners' boundaries and needs, being open to feedback and compromise, and approaching sex with an attitude of exploration and curiosity rather than judgment.

In summary, healthy sexual relationships require open communication, mutual respect, and a willingness to listen and adapt. By being transparent about needs and boundaries, promoting safe sex practices, and prioritizing mutual respect, individuals can foster supportive and empowering sexual relationships that promote overall well-being and satisfaction.

Chapter VI

Empowerment and Advocating for Inclusive Sexual Education Spaces

A. Addressing Erasure, Exclusion, and Stigmatization of Marginalized Groups

For too long, mainstream sexual education has excluded and silenced marginalized groups such as Black, Indigenous, and People of Color (BIPOC), LGBTQIA+ individuals, and those with disabilities. This has contributed to the perpetuation of damaging stereotypes, misinformation, and stigma that can harm individuals and communities.

What Is Sex

Addressing this erasure, exclusion, and stigmatization requires acknowledging and actively challenging systemic oppression. This can involve advocating for inclusive policy changes, supporting marginalized voices in the development and implementation of sexual education programs, and prioritizing a comprehensive approach to sexuality education that recognizes and respects diverse identities and experiences.

B. Overview of Different Movements

There is a growing movement towards inclusive and comprehensive sexuality education that empowers marginalized groups and expands our understanding of diverse experiences. One such approach is Comprehensive Sexuality Education (CSE), which emphasizes a holistic and rights-based approach to sexual education. This framework prioritizes such factors as gender equity, consent, bodily autonomy, healthy relationships, and sexual pleasure.

Cheryl Bach

Other movements have emerged in response to the silence and erasure experienced by various groups. For example, Black sex educators have been challenging harmful stereotypes and promoting sexual liberation within Black communities. Queer sex education centers the experiences of LGBTQIA+ individuals, recognizing the unique challenges faced by those who have been traditionally excluded from mainstream sexual education.

Disability sexuality is another area that has often been overlooked, with little information or resources available to help individuals with disabilities navigate their sexuality safely and confidently. Disability sexuality seeks to promote greater education and visibility around the diverse experiences of those with disabilities, addressing the barriers and challenges faced by this community in accessing sexual health information and resources.

C. Techniques for Creating Safe and Respectful Sexual Learning Spaces

Creating safe and respectful sexual learning spaces is essential for empowering individuals to explore their sexuality safely and confidently. Techniques for creating these spaces will depend on the specific needs and concerns of the community involved.

However, some general strategies include:

Prioritizing inclusivity: This involves recognizing and respecting diverse identities and experiences, and advocating for policies and programming that prioritize equity and inclusion.

Providing accurate and comprehensive information: This includes information on topics such as anatomy, sexuality, birth control, STIs, and consent.

Building trust: This can involve establishing a culture of respect and confidentiality, creating opportunities for individuals to ask questions and share concerns, and responding to feedback in a timely and empathetic manner.

Empowering individuals: This can involve creating opportunities for individuals to take ownership of their sexual education, and providing support and resources that enable them to make informed decisions about their sexual health.

Foster open communication: This involves creating a space where participants can feel comfortable and safe to discuss what they're experiencing and are free to ask questions. Encouraging open and honest dialogue about sex, sexuality, relationships, and more can help reduce shame and reinforce positive behaviors and beliefs.

Addressing context: Sexual education should address the broader social, cultural, and political factors that shape our understanding of sex, gender, and sexual orientation. Doing so helps to create a more holistic view of sexuality that accounts for the influence of broader social structures.

By following these strategies, educators and leaders can create safe and inclusive spaces for sexual education, negotiation, and exploration. Remember, at its core, sexual education is a compassionate and respectful communication that affirms individuals, promotes healthy relationships and fosters empowerment.

Chapter VII

Navigating Digital Sexuality

A. Exploration of Different Digital Technologies That Have Shaped Contemporary Sexuality

The rise of digital technology has dramatically changed the way we approach sex and sexuality, from online dating to virtual reality to sexting. These digital technologies offer novel ways to explore pleasure and self-discovery, providing new avenues for sexual expression and experimentation.

One significant development has been the growth of pornography, which has become more widely accessible than ever before through the internet. This has raised concerns around the impact of pornography on individuals and society, particularly with regards to sexual violence, objectification, and addiction.

Another major development has been the rise of virtual reality and sex tech, which allows individuals to simulate sexual experiences in immersive and often highly realistic environments. This has led to concerns around consent, safety, and the impact of these technologies on real-life relationships.

B. The Impacts of Social Media, Sexting, Pornography, Virtual Reality, and Other Digital Mediums on Individuals and Society as a Whole

Social media has become a significant factor in shaping modern relationships, facilitating connections between individuals across geographic and cultural boundaries. However, it has also been linked to increased pressure to present oneself in a particular way and to perform certain sexual behaviors.

Sexting, or the sharing of sexually explicit messages and images through digital means, has likewise become more widespread and accessible. While sexting can be empowering and exciting for some, it can also lead to harassment, revenge porn, and other forms of exploitation.

Pornography, as mentioned earlier, has become more widely available than ever before, with potential impacts on sexual attitudes, beliefs, and behaviors. Some studies have linked exposure to pornography to negative outcomes, including objectification, aggression, and addiction.

Virtual reality and sex tech offer exciting new opportunities for sexual exploration and pleasure, but they also raise questions around consent, safety, and the impact on relationships in the physical world. Some worry that these technologies could further isolate individuals from one another, leading to a decrease in intimacy and genuine connection.

C. Discussion of Best Practices and Safety Measures When Engaging in Digital Sexuality

Given the potential risks associated with digital sexuality, it's essential to approach these technologies with caution and mindfulness.

Here are some best practices and safety measures to consider:

Set boundaries: Establish clear boundaries around what you are comfortable sharing or viewing online and make sure your partner knows them as well.

Consent is key: Always ensure that both parties have explicit and enthusiastic consent before engaging in any sexual activity, including sexting and virtual reality experiences.

Be mindful of the impact on real-life relationships: Recognize that digital sexuality can impact your real-life relationships and take steps to ensure that these technologies don't interfere with intimacy and communication.

Consider the sources of pornography: If you choose to consume pornography, try to select sources that promote healthy and consensual sexuality.

Protect your privacy: Take measures to protect your identity and personal information online, including using secure passwords and avoiding sharing sensitive information.

Practice safe sexting: Avoid sending explicit messages or images to anyone who hasn't explicitly consented to receive them, and think carefully before sharing such content with anyone at all.

By approaching digital sexuality with mindfulness, respect for boundaries, and an emphasis on mutual consent and safety, individuals and society as a whole can navigate these technologies in a way that promotes healthy sexual expression and exploration.

Chapter VIII

Spiritual and Ritual Perspectives on Sexuality

A. Examination of Cultural and Spiritual Perspectives on Sexuality

Sexuality has played a central role in many spiritual and cultural traditions throughout history, from ancient Hinduism to contemporary Christianity. Different cultures and religions have varying views on sexuality, ranging from those which view it as sacred and holy to others which view it as sinful or shameful.

For example, in ancient Hinduism, sexuality was seen as a path to transcendence and enlightenment when approached with reverence and devotion. Tantra, a practice with roots in Hinduism and Buddhism, sees sexuality as a spiritual practice that can be used to cultivate intimacy, joy, and spiritual awakening.

In contrast, many Western religions such as Christianity and Islam view sexuality as primarily for procreation and within the bounds of heterosexual marriage. However, even within these religions, there is diversity in interpretation and practice, with some individuals and communities adopting more open and affirming attitudes towards sexuality.

B. Discussion of How Spirituality Can Influence One's Approach to Sexuality

One's personal spirituality can greatly impact their approach to sexuality and sexual expression. For example, those who view sex as a sacred act may approach it with a greater sense of reverence and mindfulness, striving to create a deeper spiritual and emotional connection with their partner.

Additionally, spirituality can influence one's values and ethics around sexuality, such as the commitment to practicing consent and respect for boundaries. Many spiritual traditions promote the values of love, compassion, and non-harm, which can be applied to sexual relationships and practices.

C. Insight into how One May Incorporate Sexuality into Spiritual Practices, Including Tantra and Ecstatic Dance

There are various ways in which individuals may incorporate sexuality into their spiritual practices, including tantra and ecstatic dance. Tantra, a spiritual practice that originated in India, incorporates sex as a means to achieve spiritual awakening and cultivate intimacy with one's partner. It emphasizes mindfulness, presence, and deep connection with oneself and one's partner.

Ecstatic dance is a form of moving meditation that aims to access altered states of consciousness, with the rhythm and music serving as a catalyst for self-expression, exploration, and transformation. In an erotic context, it can be used to tap into one's sensual energy and connect more deeply with one's body and desires.

Other rituals and practices, such as meditation, prayer, and visualization, can also be used to enhance one's sexual experiences and deepen one's connection with oneself and one's partner. By incorporating a spiritual dimension to one's sexuality, individuals can create a sense of reverence, transcendence, and meaning in their intimate lives.

However, it's important to approach these practices with caution and mindfulness. Spiritual sexuality practices should prioritize consent, communication, and respect for boundaries. It's also important to be aware of power imbalances that can arise in sexual relationships, particularly where one partner is in a position of authority or influence.

Additionally, it's worth noting that spiritual sexuality practices are not a replacement for professional therapy or medical treatment. While they can complement other forms of healing and self-exploration, they should not be used as a substitute for seeking professional help when needed.

In conclusion, spirituality and sexuality have been intertwined throughout history and across different cultures. By incorporating spirituality into our sexual practices, we can deepen our connection with ourselves and our partners and find meaning and transcendence in our intimate lives. However, we should approach these practices with mindfulness, respect for boundaries, and awareness of potential power dynamics.

Chapter IX

Conclusion and Reflections

A. Final Reflections on Comprehensive Sex Education and How It Can Impact Personal Lives and Society at Large

Comprehensive sex education is about more than just the mechanics of sex. It's about promoting healthy relationships, empowering individuals to make informed decisions about their bodies and their sexual health, and challenging harmful attitudes and behaviors that perpetuate inequality and stigma.

By providing accurate and inclusive information about sexuality, we can help individuals develop a positive and respectful relationship with their bodies and their sexuality.

Cheryl Bach

This, in turn, can lead to greater self-esteem, confidence, and sexual satisfaction.

Moreover, comprehensive sex education can have far-reaching effects for society at large. It can reduce unintended pregnancies, STIs, and sexual violence by promoting safer sex practices and respectful relationships. It can also challenge societal norms that perpetuate gender stereotypes and discrimination, leading to greater gender equality and social justice.

Overall, comprehensive sex education is an essential tool for promoting personal health and wellbeing as well as contributing to a more equitable and just society.

B. Call to Action and Activism for Better Sex Education

Despite the proven benefits of comprehensive sex education, many countries and communities have yet to fully embrace it. This can be due to a variety of reasons, such as cultural norms, political resistance, or lack of funding.

As individuals, we can take action to advocate for better sex education in our communities and beyond. This can include engaging in activism and advocacy efforts, such as contacting legislators, participating in protests, or supporting organizations that promote comprehensive sex education.

Furthermore, we can challenge stigma and misinformation around sexuality by having open and honest conversations with friends, family, and peers. By sharing accurate information and promoting respectful attitudes towards sexuality, we can help breakdown harmful stereotypes and promote a more sex-positive culture.

C. Steps Towards Discovery of Self-Love and Care

As we have seen throughout this guide, self-discovery, self-love, and self-care are central components of sexual wellness. By prioritizing care for our bodies, minds, and emotions, we can create a more positive and fulfilling relationship with our sexuality.

Some steps towards self-love and care include:

Listening to our bodies: Paying attention to our physical sensations and needs can help us better understand and respond to our own desires and boundaries.

Practicing self-compassion: Treating ourselves with kindness and understanding, especially in moments of vulnerability or self-doubt, can help us build a stronger sense of self-worth and confidence.

Exploring our desires: Experimenting with different forms of pleasure and exploring our fantasies can help us build a stronger sense of self-worth and confidence.

Cheryl Bach

www.ingramcontent.com/pod-product-compliance
Lightning Source LLC
Chambersburg PA
CBHW051705250726

48653CB00007B/2859